THE LANGUAGE OF LOVE

A Comprehensive Guide to Sex Talk

By
TERESA J. ROSE

TABLE OF CONTENTS

tion

Introduction

In a world where human connection is often reduced to emojis and fleeting messages, the realm of intimate communication remains one of the most enigmatic and uncharted territories of our lives. "The Language of Love: A Comprehensive Guide to Sex Talk" is your definitive roadmap to demystifying this intricate art and harnessing its transformative power. In these pages, we embark on an odyssey into the heart and soul of what it means to communicate intimately with our partners, igniting the fires of passion and strengthening the bonds of love.

As social beings, we are inherently wired to connect, yet many of us find ourselves stumbling through the intricate terrain of romantic and sexual communication. Whether you're in the early stages of a relationship, navigating the complexities of a long-term commitment, or embarking on a journey of self-discovery, this book serves as your trusted companion. Here, we venture beyond the superficial and delve into the profound, exploring the myriad ways in which words, gestures, and emotions converge to create a symphony of intimacy.

Chapter by chapter, we will unravel the mysteries surrounding the language of love. From the power of words and breaking down societal taboos to understanding the intricate dance of non-verbal communication, we will equip you with the tools and insights needed to cultivate a deeper, more fulfilling connection with your partner. Through open and honest discussions, we will empower you to explore your desires and boundaries, fostering an environment of trust and consent.

But our journey doesn't stop at the realms of emotional connection. We venture into the exhilarating world of seduction, teaching you the art of kindling desire, enhancing passion, and stoking the fires of longing. You'll learn to navigate the challenges that may arise on your path, from addressing sexual difficulties to embracing the liberating art of erotic communication.

In the digital age, where screens often stand between us and our partners, we examine the nuances of digital intimacy, bridging the gap between the physical and virtual worlds with grace and respect. We'll explore the depths of sensory communication, utilizing all five senses to create unforgettable, sensuous experiences that resonate in the hearts and minds of both you and your beloved.

Chapter 1

The Power of Words

In the vast landscape of human emotions and connections, words are the keystones upon which our most profound experiences are built. In the realm of intimacy, they hold an unparalleled significance, for it is through words that we not only express our desires and vulnerabilities but also establish the foundations of trust and emotional connection. Welcome to the first chapter of ***"The Language of Love: A Comprehensive Guide to Sex Talk,"*** where we will delve deep into the transformative power of words within the context of intimacy.

Understanding the Importance of Words in the Realm of Intimacy

Words have an extraordinary capacity to convey our deepest thoughts, feelings, and desires. In the context of intimacy, they become a bridge between our innermost selves and our partners. When we communicate openly and honestly, we allow our partners a glimpse into our desires, insecurities, and passions, forging a connection that transcends the physical. Through words, we have the ability to affirm our love, express our needs, and seek the understanding and validation that are fundamental to any healthy relationship. By understanding the power that words hold, we can harness this energy to enrich our connections, deepen our bonds, and create an environment where both partners feel safe and cherished.

The Role of Communication in Building Trust and Emotional Connection

Trust is the bedrock of any intimate relationship, and communication is the mortar that holds it all together. In this chapter, we will explore how effective communication builds trust and fosters emotional connection. When we express ourselves openly, honestly, and with vulnerability, we invite our partners to do the same. Through this mutual exchange, we build a sense of security, knowing that we can rely on one another to understand and support each other's needs.

Moreover, words allow us to navigate the complexities of consent and boundaries, ensuring that both partners feel respected and valued in the intimate space they share. We will discuss how clear and compassionate communication can help establish and maintain these essential aspects of a healthy sexual relationship.

Techniques for Initiating Conversations About Sex with Your Partner

Initiating conversations about sex can be daunting, but it's a crucial step in nurturing a fulfilling and satisfying intimate connection. In this section, we will provide you with practical techniques and strategies to help you broach this often sensitive topic with confidence and sensitivity.

Whether you're seeking to explore new desires, address concerns, or simply enhance your sexual experience, effective communication is the key.
We will cover the art of active listening, creating a safe and judgment-free space for dialogue, and employing empathy to understand your partner's perspective. Additionally, we will delve into the importance of timing and setting, ensuring that your discussions are conducive to productive and meaningful communication.

Chapter 2

Breaking Down Taboos

In this chapter of *"The Language of Love: A Comprehensive Guide to Sex Talk,"* we embark on a courageous journey of dismantling the societal taboos and misconceptions that have cast a shadow over our understanding of sex and intimacy. We delve deep into the heart of these issues, providing you with the tools and insights needed to break free from the shackles of shame and embarrassment, and instead, foster open and honest dialogues with your partner.

Exploring Society's Taboos and Misconceptions About Sex

Sex, despite being an integral part of the human experience, often finds itself shrouded in a veil of secrecy and misunderstanding. Society's taboos and misconceptions about sex have perpetuated myths, misinformation, and stigma that hinder our ability to communicate openly and authentically about our desires and needs.

In this section, we confront these taboos head-on, challenging the prevailing norms and beliefs that may have hindered your sexual journey. By shedding light on common misconceptions and encouraging critical thinking, we empower you to view sex as a natural, healthy aspect of human life, worthy of discussion, exploration, and celebration.

Strategies for Overcoming Shame and Embarrassment in Sexual Communication

Shame and embarrassment can be formidable barriers when it comes to discussing intimate matters with a partner. These

emotions can stem from
societal influences, personal
insecurities, or past
experiences. However, they
need not hold you back from
the enriching experience of
open communication about
sex.
In this chapter, we provide you
with practical strategies for
confronting and overcoming
these inhibitions. We will
explore methods for cultivating
self-acceptance, self-
compassion, and a positive
self-image, which are essential
for navigating the sometimes
challenging waters of sexual
conversation. Additionally,
we'll discuss the importance of
vulnerability and authenticity
in fostering a deeper
connection with your partner.

Promoting Open and Honest Dialogue with Your Partner

At the heart of this chapter lies the belief that open and honest communication is the antidote to the stigma and discomfort surrounding discussions of sex. We will guide you through the process of creating a safe and welcoming space in which both you and your partner can freely express your thoughts, feelings, and desires. Effective communication is a two-way street, and we will provide you with invaluable tools for active listening, empathy, and validation. By developing these skills, you can establish a foundation of trust and understanding that allows both you and your partner to communicate openly

without fear of judgment or
rejection.

Chapter 3

Non-Verbal Communication

In the silent eloquence of a lingering gaze, the tender brush of fingertips, and the unspoken dance of bodies, non-verbal communication in the bedroom becomes the poetic language of intimacy. In this chapter of "The Language of Love: A Comprehensive Guide to Sex Talk," we embark on a journey to explore the profound significance of body language and physical cues, offering exercises and tips to enhance your non-verbal connection with your partner. We'll delve into the art of sensuous touch and meaningful gestures, unveiling the secrets to unlocking a world of unspoken desire and connection.

The Significance of Body Language and Physical Cues in the Bedroom

Words can often falter in the face of raw passion and desire. This is where the power of body language and physical cues shines brilliantly. In the bedroom, our bodies become a canvas on which we paint the emotions and desires that words alone cannot capture. Understanding the nuances of body language allows you to decipher your partner's unspoken desires and emotions, fostering a deeper and more intuitive connection. We will explore how eye contact, posture, and subtle movements can convey longing, excitement, and affection, creating an unbreakable bond between you and your partner. Additionally, we will discuss the importance of consent and active listening in non-verbal communication, ensuring that both partners feel respected and cherished.

Exercises and Tips for Enhancing Non-Verbal Connection with Your Partner

In this section, we offer a range of exercises and practical tips designed to heighten your non-verbal connection with your partner. From mindfulness techniques that help you stay present in the moment to playful games that enhance your physical awareness, these exercises will guide you toward a deeper understanding of each other's desires and boundaries.

We will also explore the concept of mirroring, a powerful tool for building rapport and connection through non-verbal communication. By aligning your body language with your partner's, you can create a harmonious and synchronized connection that transcends words.

The Art of Sensuous Touch and Meaningful Gestures

Sensuous touch and meaningful gestures are the poetry of physical connection. They communicate love, desire, and affection in ways that words cannot. In this chapter, we will delve into the art of touch, teaching you how to use your hands, lips, and body to express passion and tenderness.

From sensual massages to gentle caresses, you will discover how to create a symphony of sensations that ignites desire and deepens emotional intimacy. Meaningful gestures, both inside and outside the bedroom, play a pivotal role in nurturing a loving connection. We will provide you with ideas and inspiration for surprise gestures that will make your partner feel cherished and adored.

Chapter 4

Exploring Desires and Boundaries

In the intricate tapestry of intimacy, desires and

boundaries are the threads that weave the fabric of a fulfilling and respectful sexual connection. ***In this chapter of "The Language of Love: A Comprehensive Guide to Sex Talk,"*** we embark on a journey through the complex landscape of sexual desires and fantasies, focusing on creating a safe space for discussing boundaries and consent. We will equip you with invaluable tools for effectively expressing your desires and, equally importantly, listening to your partner's.

Navigating the Complex Landscape of Sexual Desires and Fantasies

Our sexual desires and fantasies are as unique as our fingerprints, and yet they often remain uncharted territory within our relationships. In this section, we will guide you through the exploration of these intimate aspects of your being. We will discuss the importance of understanding your own desires and fantasies, shedding light on the fantasies that fuel your passion and excitement.

Moreover, we will address the potential disparity between your desires and your partner's, offering strategies for navigating these differences with sensitivity and respect. The goal is to create an environment where both partners feel free to express their desires and curiosities without judgment or fear.

Creating a Safe Space for Discussing Boundaries and Consent

Boundaries and consent are the cornerstones of ethical and respectful sexual relationships. In this chapter, we emphasize the critical importance of establishing and maintaining clear boundaries and enthusiastic consent within your intimate connection. We'll explore the dynamics of consent and discuss how to foster a culture of continuous, open communication in your sexual encounters.

Creating a safe space for these conversations is paramount. We will provide you with practical guidance on how to initiate discussions about boundaries and consent, ensuring that both you and your partner feel heard,

respected, and empowered in
your sexual interactions. By
fostering an environment of
trust and understanding, you
can navigate your desires and
boundaries with grace and
compassion.

Tools for Effectively Expressing Your Desires and Listening to Your Partner's

Effective communication about
desires and boundaries requires
not only the ability to express
your own needs and limits but
also the skill to listen actively
and empathetically to your
partner's. In this section, we
will equip you with tools and
techniques for these essential
aspects of sexual
communication.
You will learn how to use "I"
statements to express your

desires and boundaries in a non-confrontational manner, creating a safe and non-judgmental space for dialogue. Additionally, we will explore the art of active listening, allowing you to understand and validate your partner's feelings and boundaries.

Chapter 5

The Art of Seduction

In the dance of desire and longing, the art of seduction emerges as a tantalizing and transformative force. In this chapter of *"The Language of Love: A Comprehensive Guide to Sex Talk,"* we delve into the intricate craft of seductive communication. Whether you're in the early stages of a passionate romance or seeking

to reignite the flames of desire
in a long-term relationship,
mastering the art of seduction
can awaken your deepest
passions and build intimacy
like never before.

Mastering the Art of Seductive Communication

Seductive communication is an
art form that transcends mere
words; it is a symphony of
desire, anticipation, and allure.
In this section, we will explore
the psychology behind
seduction and provide you with
the tools to become a master
seducer. You'll learn how to
use your words, body
language, and gestures to
create an atmosphere of
irresistible attraction.
We'll also delve into the power
of anticipation, teaching you
how to kindle desire through

teasing, flirting, and the art of suggestion. By mastering these techniques, you'll become a captivating storyteller of desire, weaving a narrative that leaves your partner yearning for more.

Creating Anticipation and Excitement Through Words and Actions

Seduction thrives on anticipation and excitement. In this part of the chapter, we'll delve deeper into the role of words and actions in building desire. We'll provide you with specific language and communication techniques that can ignite the flames of passion.

You'll discover how to use text messages, notes, and even simple gestures to build anticipation and create

moments of electric
connection. We'll discuss the
importance of spontaneity and
surprise in keeping the element
of excitement alive in your
relationship.

Building Intimacy and Reigniting Passion in Long-Term Relationships

Long-term relationships can
experience periods of
complacency and routine, but
the art of seduction is a potent
elixir for rekindling passion
and intimacy. In this section,
we'll offer guidance on how to
infuse your relationship with
the vitality and allure of
seduction, even after years
together.
We'll explore how to
rediscover your partner's
desires and fantasies, creating a
sense of novelty and adventure.

You'll learn how to communicate your love and desire in ways that make your partner feel cherished and desired, renewing the emotional and physical connection between you.

Chapter 6

Talking Through Challenges

In every journey of love and intimacy, challenges and hurdles are bound to arise. In this chapter of ***"The Language of Love: A Comprehensive Guide to Sex Talk,"*** we confront these challenges head-on. We explore common sexual issues that couples often face, provide strategies for effective communication about topics such as performance

anxiety and libido differences,
and emphasize the importance
of seeking professional help
when needed, while breaking
down the stigmas surrounding
it.

Addressing Common Sexual Challenges and Issues

Sexual challenges are a natural part of the human experience, but they can sometimes be daunting to confront. In this section, we shine a light on the common sexual issues that couples encounter, including difficulties with desire, arousal, or performance. By acknowledging these challenges, you can normalize the conversation and create an atmosphere of understanding and support.

We'll provide insights into the potential causes of these issues, dispelling myths and offering guidance on how to approach them as a team. By recognizing that you're not alone in facing these challenges, you can begin to address them with empathy and compassion.

Communicating About Performance Anxiety, Libido Differences, and More

Effective communication is the key to overcoming sexual challenges. This chapter will offer you practical tips and techniques for broaching topics such as performance anxiety, differences in libido, and other common issues. We'll explore how to initiate these conversations with sensitivity and respect, ensuring that both

you and your partner feel heard
and valued.

You'll learn to create a safe and
non-judgmental space where
you can share your concerns
and vulnerabilities openly. By
fostering this environment of
trust and understanding, you'll
be better equipped to navigate
these challenges together and
find solutions that work for
both of you.

Seeking Professional Help When Needed and Breaking Down Stigmas

In some cases, professional
help may be necessary to
address sexual challenges
effectively. In this section, we
emphasize the importance of
seeking guidance from trained
therapists, counselors, or
medical professionals when
needed. We'll discuss the

benefits of professional intervention and how it can provide valuable insights and strategies for overcoming difficulties.

Additionally, we'll work together to break down the stigmas that can often surround seeking professional help for sexual issues. It's essential to recognize that reaching out for assistance is a courageous and responsible step toward enhancing your sexual well-being and the health of your relationship.

Chapter 7

Dirty Talk Done Right

In the realm of intimate communication, there exists a seductive and powerful language that transcends the ordinary: the art of dirty talk. In this chapter of ***"The Language of Love: A Comprehensive Guide to Sex Talk,"*** we explore the psychology behind erotic communication. We'll teach you the delicate craft of crafting sensual and arousing messages for your partner and provide tips for incorporating dirty talk into your intimate moments, enhancing your connection on a profound and sensual level.

The Psychology Behind Erotic Communication

Dirty talk is a captivating blend of psychology and passion. In this section, we delve into the psychological underpinnings of erotic communication. We'll discuss the role of verbal and non-verbal cues in arousal, exploring how words can stimulate desire, anticipation, and excitement. Understanding the psychology behind dirty talk is crucial for appreciating its potential to enhance intimacy and pleasure. We'll shed light on how it can boost confidence, increase emotional connection, and ignite the fires of passion in the bedroom.

Crafting Sensual and Arousing Messages for Your Partner

The art of crafting sensual and arousing messages requires finesse and creativity. In this part of the chapter, we'll provide you with practical guidance on how to choose the right words, tone, and timing for your messages. You'll learn to tap into your partner's desires and fantasies, creating a dialogue that resonates with their deepest longings. We'll explore various techniques for crafting dirty talk messages, from the subtle and suggestive to the bold and explicit, allowing you to customize your communication to match your partner's preferences and comfort level. By mastering this art, you can evoke desire and pleasure like never before.

Tips for Incorporating Dirty Talk into Your Intimate Moments

Dirty talk is a versatile tool that can be woven seamlessly into your intimate moments. In this section, we offer tips and strategies for incorporating erotic communication into your sexual encounters. We'll discuss the importance of consent and open communication with your partner to ensure that dirty talk enhances rather than detracts from your shared experiences.

You'll also gain insights into creating a comfortable and non-judgmental space for dirty talk, where both you and your partner feel free to express your desires and fantasies without inhibition. By mastering the art of timing and delivery, you can build anticipation and excitement, taking your intimacy to new heights.

Chapter 8

Beyond Words - Sensory Communication

In the intimate realm of love and desire, there exists a profound language that transcends speech and words—a language of sensation and emotion. In this chapter of "The Language of Love: A Comprehensive Guide to Sex Talk," we embark on a journey into the world of sensory communication in the bedroom. We explore the ways in which the senses of sight, sound, smell, taste, and touch can enhance intimacy, leading to unforgettable sensual experiences that deepen your connection with your partner.

Exploring the World of Sensory Communication in the Bedroom

Sensory communication is a dance of heightened awareness and profound connection. In this section, we delve into the sensory landscape of the bedroom, where the senses become your most powerful tools for creating intimacy. We'll explore how each of the five senses contributes to your sensual experience, from the allure of sight to the evocative power of touch. By understanding how sensory communication operates in the bedroom, you can harness the full spectrum of sensations to build a deeper and more enriching connection with your partner.

Enhancing Intimacy Through Sight, Sound, Smell, Taste, and Touch

The senses are gateways to heightened arousal and emotional connection. In this part of the chapter, we provide you with insights and techniques for enhancing intimacy through each of the senses.

Sight: Discover how lighting, visual stimuli, and the art of anticipation can create a visually enticing experience that awakens desire.

Sound: Explore the role of soundscapes, whispers, and vocalization in stimulating the senses and deepening emotional connection.

Smell: Dive into the world of aphrodisiac scents and the power of pheromones in igniting passion and desire.

Taste: Delve into the pleasures of sensual cuisine and the art of tantalizing the palate to heighten intimacy.

Touch: Learn how to use tactile sensations, from feather-light caresses to more assertive touches, to build a sensual and emotional connection that resonates on a profound level.

Creating Unforgettable Sensual Experiences

The culmination of sensory communication lies in the creation of unforgettable sensual experiences. In this section, we explore how to weave together the threads of sight, sound, smell, taste, and touch to craft moments of profound intimacy and pleasure.

We'll guide you through the art of sensory exploration, offering ideas and inspiration for sensory-rich encounters that leave a lasting imprint on your relationship. These experiences are not only sensual but deeply emotional, fostering a connection that transcends the boundaries of everyday life.

Chapter 9

The Language of Love in the Digital Age

In an era defined by technology and connectivity, our understanding of love and intimacy has evolved to encompass the digital realm. In this chapter of ***"The Language of Love: A Comprehensive Guide to Sex Talk,"*** we embark on a journey to navigate the intricacies of love and intimacy in the digital age. We'll explore how to navigate sexting, online dating, and long-distance relationships, balance virtual intimacy with real-life connections, and ensure that your digital interactions maintain privacy and respect.

Navigating Sexting, Online Dating, and Long-Distance Relationships

The digital age has reshaped the landscape of romantic and sexual relationships. In this section, we delve into the world of sexting, online dating, and long-distance love. We'll provide you with insights on how to navigate these modern forms of connection, from crafting engaging and flirty messages to building meaningful online relationships.

Whether you're looking to spice up your sexting game, explore the world of online dating, or maintain a loving connection with a partner who is miles away, we'll offer tips and strategies to help you thrive in the digital realm.

Balancing Virtual Intimacy with Real-Life Connections

While digital communication can offer unique avenues for connection, it's essential to strike a balance between virtual intimacy and real-life connections. In this part of the chapter, we'll explore the art of blending online and offline experiences. We'll discuss how to nurture the emotional connection built through digital interactions and translate it into physical intimacy. Whether you're transitioning from online dating to a real-world encounter or maintaining a long-distance relationship, we'll provide guidance on how to keep the flames of passion alive when you're together and apart.

Safeguarding Your Privacy and Maintaining Respect in the Digital Realm

In the digital age, privacy and respect are paramount. In this section, we'll emphasize the importance of safeguarding your personal information and maintaining respect in your digital interactions. We'll discuss how to protect your privacy online, from secure messaging apps to setting boundaries and managing your digital footprint.

Respectful communication in the digital

realm is crucial for building healthy relationships. We'll explore how to communicate effectively, set expectations, and establish boundaries with your online connections to ensure that your interactions are respectful and consensual.

Chapter 10

Keeping the Flame Alive

The final chapter of our journey in ***"The Language of Love: A Comprehensive Guide to Sex Talk"*** brings us to a crucial destination – sustaining the flames of passion and connection throughout the course of your relationship. In this chapter, we explore the art of keeping the flame alive by sustaining passionate communication, evolving your sexual communication over time, and reigniting the spark even when faced with challenges.

Sustaining Passionate Communication Throughout the Course of a Relationship

As relationships mature, maintaining the spark of passion can be a delightful challenge. In this section, we delve into the importance of sustaining passionate communication throughout your journey together. We'll explore how love and intimacy evolve over time and the role of open and honest communication in keeping the connection alive.

You'll discover strategies for expressing your love, desire, and appreciation as your relationship progresses. By continually expressing your affection and desire, you'll create an atmosphere of romance and connection that deepens over the years.

Strategies for Evolving and Adapting Your Sexual Communication Over Time

Sexual communication is not static; it evolves and adapts as your relationship matures. In this part of the chapter, we provide you with guidance on how to evolve your sexual communication to match the changing dynamics of your partnership. We'll discuss how to navigate life transitions, from parenthood to career changes, while maintaining a strong and vibrant sexual connection. You'll learn to adapt to the shifting sands of desire, explore new fantasies and desires together, and develop communication skills that grow and strengthen as your love deepens.

Reigniting the Spark Even in the Face of Challenges

Challenges are inevitable in any relationship, but they need not extinguish the flame of passion. In this section, we explore how to reignite the spark even in the face of adversity. Whether you're dealing with stress, health issues, or any other challenges that life throws your way, we'll provide you with practical strategies for keeping the fire of desire burning bright. We'll discuss the importance of emotional connection during tough times and how to use communication to deepen your bond and reignite the passion that brought you together in the first place.

Conclusion

"The Language of Love: A Comprehensive Guide to Sex Talk" has taken you on a profound and transformative journey into the realm of intimate communication. Throughout this book, we've explored the intricate art of verbal and non-verbal expression in matters of the heart and body, providing you with the tools and insights needed to deepen your connection with your partner, experience greater satisfaction, and nurture a love that grows even more profound with each passing day.

As you close the final chapter of this guide, you stand ready to embark on a voyage that will forever change the way you speak the language of love. Armed with knowledge, understanding, and a newfound confidence in your ability to communicate openly and authentically about love, desire, and intimacy, you are now equipped to foster a stronger and more fulfilling connection with your partner. Remember that the journey of love is a lifelong one, and the language of love is one that evolves and adapts over time. Whether you are in the early stages of a passionate romance or have shared many years together, the principles and techniques you've gained from this guide will continue to serve you well. The key lies in the ongoing commitment to nurturing your intimate connection, maintaining open and honest communication, and exploring the depths of desire and emotion with your beloved.

As you move forward on your journey, may your love flourish, your desires be fulfilled, and your connection grow ever stronger. May you continue to speak the language of love with eloquence, passion, and authenticity, creating a bond that is truly extraordinary.

Thank you for joining us on this profound exploration of intimacy and communication. Your dedication to enhancing your relationships and your commitment to speaking the language of love are truly commendable. Here's to a future filled with deeper connections, boundless passion, and a love that knows no bounds.